I0417346

Walking in South Lanzarote

Lanzarote

Lanzarote may be the most dramatic and exciting venue we have found. Though hot, it is breezy and perfectly comfortable for walking. The landscape is unlike anything in the world and a few minutes walking away from the car is rewarded far more than can possibly be imagined. To top a volcano's corona and gaze inside is an experience not to be missed and never to be forgotten.

We are...

Alan is the brains of the operation; Neil is the chronicler. Alan knows nearly every path on the island and either he accompanies the acolytes or directs the walk from a distance. I put it onto paper.

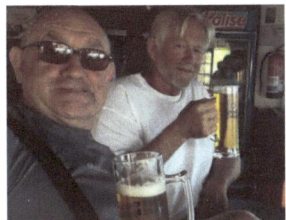

It always starts in Reiners Bar, with a couple of Estrella *'Dos jarra pour favour.'* Remember that one; you'll need it if you are going to join us on walks.

It sometimes starts goes, *'Be ready at nine, tomorrow, if you can. I've got a walk planned'.* That presages a cracking good outing.

Or else it's, *'Here's a walk you might like'.* That means I'm going alone. Good fun, but I'll get lost.

Then there's Emma. She accompanies me whenever she can, mostly because she thinks Neil shouldn't be let allowed out alone. I expect she's right; she usually is. And Wendy, whose blog and kindness have made everything possible.

> *'It's really fun to be striving to pick out a route to the top of the mountain, or to follow a map, or to decipher the ravings of a walking guide author. The work is hard but you don't notice because the barranco is exciting or the mountain path thrilling and then suddenly you reach the corona and look down in awe into the bowl of another volcano, or you struggle to the peak and admire the view of the whole world.'*

Note: This text is offered on the inventive new 'Createspace' Publishing platform for two reasons:

1) The costs to the reader are far lower than traditional publishing houses.
2) It is easy to update and improve the work; the text is continually under review. To this end the readers and the authors form a community to develop the work. As a reader, you are invited to email suggestions to nwheeler@brookes.ac.uk Contributions may be simple 'typo' alerts, corrections to detail, new areas to cover, etc. All contributors are acknowledged in the print and E-Book versions, with our thanks.

Contents

Join us…

For our first five years visiting Lanzarote I believed that lying on a sun-bed was of itself exhausting enough and to arise and walk to the pool was a heroic achievement worthy of universal approbation. Walking for any distance was right out!

For the last few years, though, I've found that that is not entirely so. Egged on by Alan I've walked up endless mountains and marvelled at island views and the insides of volcanoes. The view from some of the cliffs and coronas is breath-taking *(although, admittedly that could just be the walk to reach them)*. A side effect of this exercise is that it has resolved the problem of dampness in my wardrobe. Previously, I found that the trousers I wore to fly to Lanzarote would shrink in the wardrobe and prove too small to wear for the return trip. Since I started walking, I have found the *'shrinking in the wardrobe'* problem wholly alleviated. Sometimes they are too big! Bring a belt.

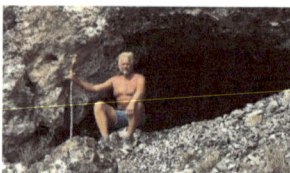 I am not learned with regard to Lanzarote after fewer than ten years. But I know a man who is. Alan has been my walking mentor in person and by remote instruction for some time. 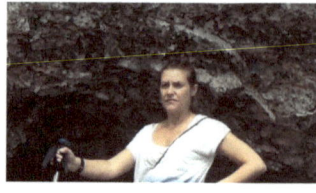 This guide reports on Alan's instruction and my slow learning journey to progressively understand and appreciate an island that has me completely captivated. If you use it you will not learn from me, but you might learn something with me. As I observe and wonder, I enquire and find out. If you walk with me, we will be discovering Lanzarote together.

On walking guides…

Walking guides come in many forms, and it is *'horses for courses'*. Some are written by professional writers who have been granted enough expenses for a week in a resort and write excellent prose about their limited 'finds'. This will suit the short-visit tourist adequately but walks tend to be basic, without the little diversions that make them exciting. Another model is the *'back-of-my-hand'* local enthusiast who will know every twisty turn, diversion and staggering view in the locality and describe them for you as well as he/she can. This well suits the adventurous walker who wants the best and doesn't mind deciphering opaque explanations and still getting lost. When you know something very well it's easy to assume rather than explain. Some fine guides endeavour to combine both, in a rich compromise.

This guide is certainly not better or worse than those approaches; just different. It will suit some readers. The intention is for the reader to explore a fantastic island alongside the author. As I discover, I report so that you can find it, too. You might learn about Lanzarote alongside me, but not from me.

> *And roughly, as a guide, anything in italics in this book can be skipped over – probably best that you do.*

On litter…

Self-evidently, walkers enjoy and respect the countryside and do not leave litter, so this book does not exhort you to *'take it home'*. However, for myself I go one step further. It is my practice to take 4-cent carrier bag on every walk and set myself the target of filling it with cans, bottles and plastics, before the end of the walk. Sadly, this is not a difficult challenge. Patently, one old chap with a carrier bag will not make a dent in Lanzarote's litter problem, but it is good to feel that you left it better than you found it if only slightly. As guests in an unbelievable landscape perhaps it behoves us to make a positive contribution, be it never so small.

On safety...

I don't really like heights, but I walk up mountains and down cliffs. If vertigo is an issue for you *(as it is for me)*, it might be because of the odd perspective you get from and each level seeming to move differently as you walk. This is a problem of parallax. I'm a height wimp, so I find it good to watch my feet when walking and stand dead still when I want to admire the view.

Winds can be extreme on Lanzarote and it is radically different on different parts of the island. On occasion we have decided not to get out of the car at all, so badly was the wind rocking it. All mountain peak, corona or cliff walks should be seen as out of bounds on a windy day.

Don't run out of light. Dusk this near the equator is brief; it goes dark fast! So check the sundown time and allow a big margin for error when planning an outing.

All of these walks have been extensively tested; we find them safe enough – for us. By the time you read it, things can have changed, because of rain, rock falls, erosion or whatever. And your agility might be different from ours, so you must judge the safety of every enterprise you understate. We are not saying that any walk is safe today or for you, only that it was safe when we did it, for us. We cannot accept responsibility for your misfortune that occurs on your walk. You walk at your own risk!

And health...

This walking lark is worth it for the breath-taking views but to make it healthy they recon you need to be a little breathless on the ascents but still able to hold a conversation. *(Mind you that last bit always looks a bit dodgy when I walk alone.)* Carry sun block and lip-balm for regular application, especially if you're not well thatched. Carry copious water. Sometimes I don't get thirsty at all and the next time, a litre is gone in no time. Possibly we are affected by humidity. When the air is very dry and whipping past on a hot day it does seem to rip the water out of you.

Blisters happen so carry plasters. I also carry a spare pair of shoes and socks, as different from the ones I am walking in as possible. That means that if a shoe is rubbing I can put on another pair that does not have the same pressure points. Wear sun protecting clothes.

A compass and map will get you home wherever you are and a whistle is good in the event that you want to attract attention. Signal is pretty good so take a 'phone and know where you are should you need to summon aid. There is only one really good map: 'Lanzarote Tour and Trail'. It's not in many shops here, so Google it!

On paths...

I use the term 'path' rather loosely in places. Some are thin but clear, sometimes they vanish without warning. I find that if the path vanishes, it's because I've wondered off it. If I stop and look around I usually spot it and return is easy. Sometimes it just peters out. Then it is good to have Hiawatha with you. If you can see trainer prints every now and then you are probably still on the route.

Sometimes you realise that it is not a path, but a goat trail; sometimes it is a rain gulley (Barranco).

There are also *'Hogwarts paths'* that can be clear as day from a distance but when you reach them and try to follow them, they will completely vanish. Lanzarote *'Hogwart's paths'* appear and disappear at will. I personally think that they do so simply to inconvenience walkers.

Jerome K Jerome says of kettles, 'one must pretend to take no notice of it, if you want it to boil. It is a good plan, too, to talk loudly about how you don't feel like tea and will not drink any of it when it's ready and would really prefer lemonade.'

I find the same works for some paths. If I say 'look for path A' or 'Take track B' you will not find either in a month of weekends. If we pretend not to care about paths at all, then one will pop up in no time. Just until it thinks you are beginning to like following it and then it will instantly vanish. I tried a good trick on one. When I stumbled upon it I turned and followed it backwards for that way it was as clear as day. The path was happy to be followed as long as it thought it was leading me in the wrong direction. Before long it smelled a rat, though, and realized that I was liking following it so 'Poof!' it was gone.

So, we give out that we do not want to use the path anyway. One day we are on a 'path unlooked for' and we follow it for a bit loudly saying things like, 'I'm not bothered about this path either way. Are you, Emma?' 'No not me; I'm happy keeping the mountain on my left elbow; don't need a path at all, really. Aren't you the same, Neil?' 'Oh, yes, that's good enough for me; I've no use for a path.' Keeping this up means that the path continues for some way before it cottons on to our ruse and then 'Poof!' It is Gone.

Anyway, each walk is independently pilot tested to assure me that the description works, so you should be OK, and even if you are unable to find a trail (maybe it was washed away) it's a small island and a road always appears before long.

On equipment…

A compass and a map make a good start. That way, you'll find a route under any circumstances. More importantly, when you reach a peak, you're surrounded by views over a range of villages, mountains and 'whatnot' and it is great fun to sit and identify each from the map. There is only one really good map: 'Lanzarote Tour and Trail'. It's not in many shops here, so Google it!

Some people like to walk in heavy hiking boots, but for most of these walks, walking trainers are enough. Only where walking is over very rocky lava would a hard sole be advisable to prevent metatarsal bruising. The walk guide will warn you.

I take spare footwear, as different from what I have on my feet as possible. If I get a blister, I can change into something with different pressure points. Sandalss, for instance mean that blistered toes are safe.

Water is crucial. Decide how much you need for the number of hours that you will walk and double it. On some occasions, when the wind is strong and the humidity very low, water loss can be quite remarkable. An ice cold beer is recommended in many of the walks but that's not always the best way to re-hydrate. Take plenty of water before starting on the Estrella.

Take sun cream for periodic reapplying and protective headwear, *(especially if you are folically challenged as is one of the authors).*

A stick has two benefits.

Firstly, on some walks the ground is unsteady because gravel and stones can move underfoot. A third point of contact can be a life-saver when the ground slips and your feet go out from under you. My stick has saved me on many occasions.

Secondly, in terms of exercise value, using a stick is an upper limb workout to complement your lower limb exercise. Alternate hands and you will develop muscle evenly.

Just occasionally, you might be pleased that have lightweight raingear in your backpack. When it rains in Lanzarote, it doesn't mess around!

Flora and fauna

Far more grows on the island than people imagine; the soil is very much more fertile that it appears and water can be taken from the humid atmosphere by cunning deployment of pecon. Farming includes: Lanzarote palms, grapes, figs, olives, orange, lemon, almonds, potatoes, leeks, onions, peas, strawberries, melons, chillies and peppers, etc (and etc!). The fresh food offer with minimal food miles is quite remarkable.

Wild plants include a wealth of cacti, geraniums, sedum, nicotiana, and many more. After a little rain, the island hosts masses of wild-flower meadows.

In the sky, there are hawks, kestrels, buzzards, ravens, little egrets, choughs, sparrows, hoopoes, doves, pipits, chaffinches, goldcrests, canaries and more. **On the ground** there are lizards and their heavier cousins, geckoes. These will eat banana from your hand in many of the beachside pods. There are mice, rabbits and hedgehogs everywhere if you look for the signs. **In the sea** there is an incredible array of fish.

Places to visit

For us, the island is unrivalled in the world for landscape and artefacts and it rewards a trip out by car when you are showing the unquestionable wisdom of declining to walk up a mountain. The following is a basic list and we generally don't like visitors to leave until they have experienced each of them at least once. As an economy, it is possible to buy a batch of tickets allowing entry to five of these remarkable locations at a significant reduction – and well worth it.

The Cactus Garden.

Guatiza on the LZ1 hosts this amazing garden. The layout is extremely clever and the collection of cacti breath-taking. A look inside the windmill is also a privilege. Nearby, in Mala, there is the renowned Arepera Restaurant and across the main road from there it is possible to see *(from the road and for free)* an almost better cactus garden; check out both on one trip.

Jamos Del Aqua.

This staggering cave system is on the LZ1 Orzola Road is a most amazing experience, not to be missed, but frequently to be repeated *(we do, anyway)*.

Cueva los Verda.

Another cave system, actually linked to *Jamos Del Aqua,* being part of the same lava tube, is just off the LZ1 Orzola road on the LZ204. This is a very different but equally amazing experience, also not to be missed.

The Mirador Del Rio.

This Mirador (viewing point) is near Orzola on the North-West extreme of the island and is a magnificent Cesar Monrique construction. After enjoying the building and the view for a bit, I have to marvel about how they built it.

Salinas de Janubio

On the South-West coast, not far from Playa Blanca is an active salt pan, where hills of salt are to be seen. There is an intriguing system of canals designed to take sea water and fill each bay where it is left to evaporate and the salt collected by hand. This pan is still said to produce 15,000 tonnes of salt per year, but that is less than a third of production of this industry in its heyday. Before, refrigeration, the salt was a major industry for the island, being used to preserve fish. Today's harvest is exported. *(There being little need to salt the roads in Lanzarote.)*

Fuego de Timanfaya.

The famous, Fire Mountain, on the west of the island is a true spectacle. Ideally visit at opening time (10-am) because the access is narrow and traffic builds up later in the day. The crust is thin and ground too hot in places to walk. See geysers, barbeque meat over the hot ground and take the bus tour over a landscape that you will never forget.

Los Hevidaros

This is a fabulous spectacle on the West coast, on the LZ702 that sees crashing waves assault the cliff and pass under natural arches and you can watch it all from walkways and galleries built into and on top of the cliff. This is unlike anything else on the island. Like so much else that is good on Lanzarote the layout was designed by Cesar Monrique.

El Golfo.

On the West coast, on the LZ702 lies this is a charming village and a short walk *(No, Really; it is a very short walk)* over a hill takes you to an emerald green inland lake. There are a few nice restaurants, too.

The two homes of Cesar Monrique,

Both of Monrique's homes were donated to become museums. One is in Haria and the other (The Foundation) is near to Tahiche. Both need to be seen *(to be believed)*. They represent eccentricity at its most brilliant.

Lag Omar,

In Nazaret near Teguise, signed from the LZ10, Lag Omar is a home built by Cesar Monrique for Omar Sharif. It is set into a quarry rock face with external staircases linking normal rooms, each build into a cave. The surreal placing of (for example) modern kitchen fittings into a cave is something that will blow you away.

Castillo Santa Barbara

Is a castle near to the old capital town, Teguise, where it was once necessary to retreat from pirates; a dramatic building with far reaching views. A few minutes' study here will give a real insight into the lives of islanders plagued by pirates.

Wine and cheese, unspoiled Bodega

Leaving Orzola heading South-Westerly on the LZ201, you may be lucky enough to see a hand painted sign on your right for this Mexican style farm. Drive in for charming wine and cheese tasting in a building that might be a living museum. This is much more 'real' *(not to say cheaper)* than the big commercial wineries that you would find in La Garia.

Lanzarote a Caballo

To be found on the LZ2 near Playa del Carmen the Lanzarote a Caballo offers pony and camel riding in a very nice and informal way. You can ride camels at the Fuego de Timanfaya, but that is a little *coach-trippy*. For a far more personal experience riding on a saddle not in a basket, go to Cabello. If you prefer, they would arrange horse riding, buggies, trikes, and even paint ball (if you must). 10:00 AM to 05:30 PM.

Beaches

Playa de Papagayo, near Playa Blanca is a great place to play in the waves on a sandy beach and affords plenty of scope for sandcastles. One beach is clothed; one beach is naturist. You can take your pick.

Playa de Famara on the West coast is a long sandy beach great for views and sun with a naturist tolerance, but although there are surfers galore, it is not recommended for swimming as the currents are dangerous and drownings are recorded almost every year.

Orzola and Isla Graciosa. At the northern extremity of the island, on the LZ1 Orzola has the ferry to Isla Graciosa which has some very fine beaches. Heading North on the LZ1, approaching Orzola there are several small isolated sandy places by the water with parking allowing secluded bathing and Orzola itself has a good safe beach.

Towns

See: Haria, Teguise, Yaiza, Uga and Femes if nowhere else, but really the style of house and their general unspoiled nature makes all of the old towns a treat to visit. *(The new ones, of course, are rather a matter of taste.)*

Markets

Arrecife   Monday to Friday:
Recova Market 9am to 2pm - Fresh local produce and local artisan craft shops
Fish Market - 9am to 1pm - Local fish and sea food caught fresh each day
Playa Blanca   Wednesday & Saturday
Marina Rubicon - 9.30am to 1.30pm - About 30 stalls with crafts, jewellery, arts and books
Costa Teguise Friday
Pueblo Marinero - 6pm to 10pm - Small and busy evening market, mainly crafts and souvenirs, great atmosphere.
Haria   Saturday
Artisan Market - 10am to 2.30pm - Various stalls with handmade crafts and artwork, some local produce stalls, a bit quirky and different.
Tias   Saturday
Recova Market - 9am to 2pm - Small market with local goods and produce

Mancha Blanca Sunday
Local agricultural market- 9am to 2pm - The best island market for local produce and fresh fruit and vegetables.
Teguise   Sunday
Island market - 9am to 2pm - The biggest market in Lanzarote selling everything; arts, jewellery, clothes, bags, linen and leather goods.

El Golfo Montana Quemada Playa Del Paso Circle

This is a 3-hour, hard soled boot walk, not strenuous, with no risk of vertigo, in spite of a 148m peak height. Fine views.

Take a compass, binoculars a map and your stick.

Not remote. This is one of those walks that take us over well-trodden paths where your heart-attack will see you discovered and revived in mere minutes. We prefer *the path less trodden* where when you are eventually found it will be no more than your bleached bones that remain to decorate the scenery, but this is none such.

We drive to El Golfo on LZ704 and park in the large car park on the left. We walk back up the LZ704 until we see a track on the Left with a rubbish bin.

We follow the track marvelling at how it was built. The larva is so rough that it can hardly be walked and tracked vehicles could not cross it. It amazes me how roads are built through that terrain.

We continue, curving right at a farm, pausing only to pat the donkey, and continue until reaching a turning on the left with a remarkable and wholly incongruous gateway. Pause to wonder why it is here, and then pass through. A few yards further on we take a faint path right, uphill through the pecon

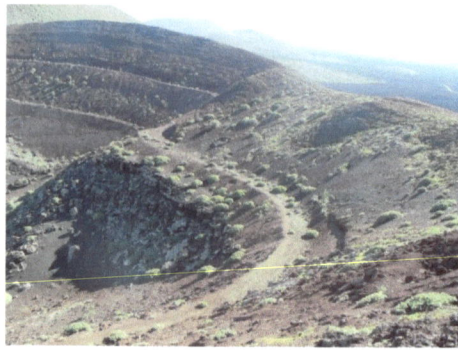

passing stone enclosures, marvelling at how these lava stones lock together in the weakest looking structures but form imperishable structures all over the island.

Suddenly topping the ridge, we fain interest in the view to gain time to recover our breath. In fact the view into the volcano is spectacular and the views backwards show El Golfo and the sea to good effect. *(Nothing to the sea views that are to come, though.)*

We ascend to the peak on our left, to experience the full view and then follow a faint path down to a track half way down the slope. We might pop down to the basin and back up, or not as we decide at the time.

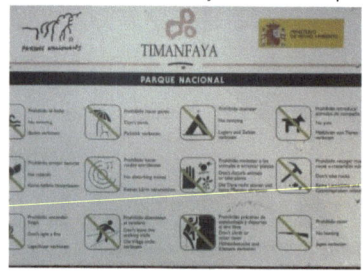

Follow the track to the left, towards a farm house. Keep to the right, so as not to encroach on the house, and we walk past his windmill and down through the pecon to avoid trespassing on his garden. Then back onto the track, passing a national park symbol and a brilliant: *'Do Not..'* sign. This one is so comprehensive as to impress, even on Lanzarote. Essentially, you are not allowed to do anything at all. Nothing! Not even a few things! Whatever you have in mind – don't do it! .

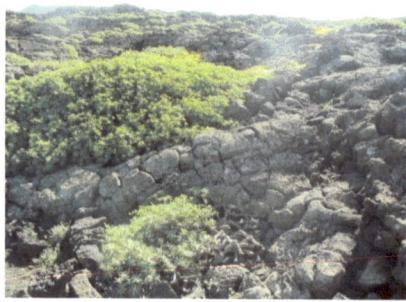

Follow this road; it's a good way but easy walking, until you reach a lovely cove with a black sand beach under a most impressive volcanic cliff. This is a great place for our snack and maybe a quick dip. Didn't bring a costume? Well, it's pretty secluded.

We return back up the track until we reach a sign with a map of this part of the national park. Take a path on our right (South) through the lava to see terrain we will just never find anywhere else. The path is well marked, but rough, so we're pleased we wore hard soled boots. The ground is up and down all of the way and the reason is that we are going over an endless series of lava tubes, measuring from ½-metre up to 10-meters in diameter. In places we can see openings that look like vaulted entrances to a man-made structure. In places we see long tubes, weaving, snaking and dividing on the surface. In places the tube is broken open and we can see it running both ways. In places, larger tubes open up to make remarkable cave systems, although as this is National Park, we're not really supposed to leave the track to explore them.

The path runs close to the edge of the cliff and the sea view is really dramatic. Also we are looking right down onto our beach of earlier. How do you feel about that *'skinny dipping'* now?

The path is a fascinating walk, with things you'll not see elsewhere, but it's hard going and continues for an hour or more, so when we return to the village, and find ½-doz fine restaurants offering us our usual post-perambulatory cold beer, we don't hesitate. The sea view is pleasant, so this makes a good time to reminisce and swear that this time we really will be strong and refuse to take any more of these crazy walks.

Continuing on to the end of the village returns us to the car that we left when we so unwisely decided to walk off up the hill.

> You know, we only undertook this walk, years ago, because we were all feeling a bit seedy. One of us had a bad knee and giddiness so that he hardly knew what he was doing. The next also had giddiness and hardly knew what she was doing, either. With me, it was liver. I knew it was liver because I had been reading the symptoms on a patent medicine packet and I found that I had them all. It is an extraordinary thing that I have never yet seen a patent medicine advertisement without realizing that I have all of the symptoms described. I think they must target these advertisements terribly well.

> I did wonder if it was just clever advertising; but, No. When I looked in a medicine book of the highest repute, I found that indeed it is true; I do have all of those diseases and a good many more besides. It can seem a bit dispiriting to have so many life-threatening problems but if you are careful then the thoroughness of your investigation takes over and your imminent demise from innumerable causes seems to get lost in the exciting study of it all. I found that the Diphtheria was going to be one cause of my eventual failure, but that the yellow fever although classic in its symptomology was in such a mild form that I could survive it for many years if properly controlled.

> Anyway, we all thought that exercise and fresh sea air would be just the thing, so we soon found ourselves struggling up the volcano and down to the sea. I'm pretty much cured, but I do find that the others are a bit giddy yet and I'm quite of the view that they rarely know where they are. *(With apologies to Gerome)*

The Secret garden

This is a 2-hour, there-and-back, trainers, walk. Easy to find, with strenuous hill sections followed by restful descents, and jolly good for you it is, too! There's no risk of vertigo, in spite of a 100-m height cliff. Fine sea views, and creations, quixotic even by Lanzarote standards.

Bring a memento to leave at the garden. Take a compass, binoculars a map and your stick.

Quite remote, in places. Some walks take us over well-trodden paths where your heart-attack will see you discovered and revived in mere minutes. We love this one because it takes us on *the path less travelled* and when you are eventually found it will be no more than your bleached bones remaining to decorate the scenery.

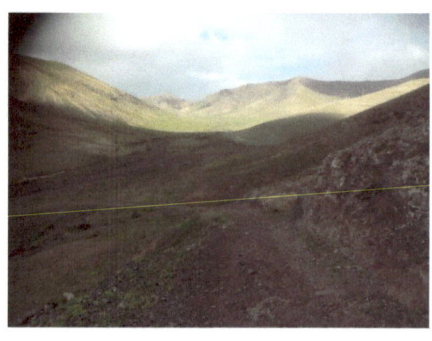

Take the LZ2, south and turn left at the Lanzarote safari roundabout onto the LZ706 to reach   Playa Quemada village on the East coast, two villages South of Puerto Del Carmen. We park on Calle el Toscon, at the South end of the village and walk South.

Leave the village following the coastal path South, zig-zagging up the hill to the crest. This is a slog, and you should be breathless but just able to talk if you are to benefit from it.

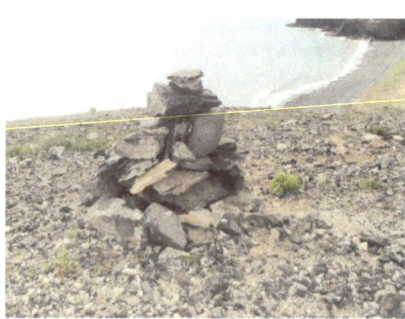

Observe the many stone cairns along the way. Some say that these delineate land boundaries and others that they mark the path. My theory is that each commemorates somebody who died on one of Alan's more strenuous walks.

From the top, take time to recover under the guise of appreciating the fine view over a deep-blue sea. Further out to sea we can see the large net enclosures and pontoons of the tuna fish farm. We walk down into the valley, where there is a pleasant black sand beach. At low tide we could have walked to this point on the beach; at high tide - not so much.

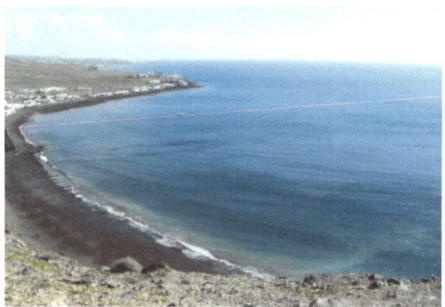
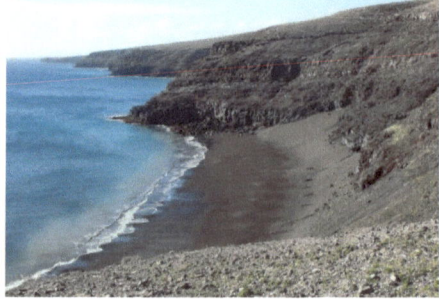

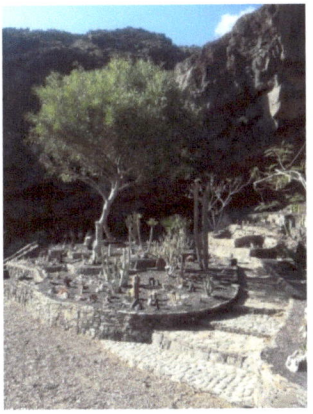

We then zig-zag up the next hill. This *effort-followed-by-easy-walking* repeated cycle is doing you the power of good! We cross a barranco and then a second descent takes us to another large beach. Here there are a good range of ruined buildings worth a few moments' study, before we struggle up the next hill.

We cross two more barrancos noticing that they exit the cliff at least 50-metres above the sea. In the rain *(and rain it does!)* the water spouts must be a sight to see. We then drop down to the next cove and are just astounded by what we find.

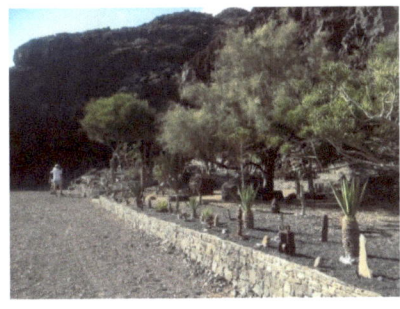

Stop here to eat and drink, and maybe leave a memento to prove that you were foolish enough to undertake this walk and visit the garden. You'll see that many people have done that. This is a nice pebbly beach, secluded in places, so a dip is not out of the question.

Finally, you can retrace your steps. Oddly enough, it is never so far when you are going back. There are restaurants offering us our usual post-perambulatory cold beer. The sea view is pleasant, so this makes a good time to reminisce and swear that this time we really will be strong and refuse to take any more of these crazy walks. Maybe we should sign the pledge, now.

I the undersigned,

(insert name here)

In the company of those present, do pledge that nevermore will I be persuaded to undertake a Lambert & Wheeler Walk. I will withstand threats and inducements and hold resolute to this oath until the day I weaken.

(Sign here)

Witnesses:

(All those present sign here)

Femés: better than the Mirador.

This is a ½-hour, up and back, trainers walk, easy to find, with one hard hill sections followed by a fabulous view and restful if picky descent. There is no risk of vertigo, despite remarkable views of the South and West of the island.

If it's not too windy, you have a spare 1/2 –hour and want to see the West coast and the Playa Blanca plain as never before, trot up this little hill and back. Take a compass, binoculars a map to help identify what you see and also your stick.

Taking the LZ702 to Femés, we park outside of the eponymous Femes Café. Where we will take coffee, now, and stew later while benefiting from clean toilets.

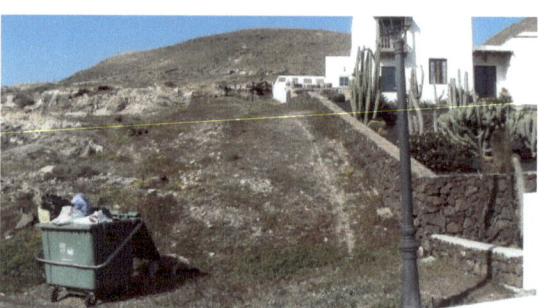

From the Church head uphill, passing the signed Mirador and turn Right onto a brick paved road. Very soon there is a rubbish bin on the Left and a 'path' running up between the bin and a garden wall. Our task is to head to the apex of this little mound. We must not be deterred by the rapid failure of any path; the direction is easy and clear. It may take up to 15-minutes and a good few calories to reach the top. As we top the mound, the entire West coast is suddenly revealed, to the most dramatic effect. The view to the south is also dramatic, looking down onto the Mirador, far below, the entire Playa Blanca plain and then the ocean.

Stay and Marvel and then return to the village. We particularly recommend the eponymous Café Femés, for beer and goat stew. It will also be a good place to congratulate yourselves on taking the shortest of the many walks starting from Femes.

Femés short, West loop for the intrepid

This is a 1½-hour, circular, trainers walk, mostly easy to find, with one or two hard hill sections followed by restful descents through rough terrain with unreliable paths but clear direction. There's no great risk of vertigo, and remarkable views of the South and West of the island. This is a nice walk around the edge of this very charming town. Take a compass, binoculars a map and your stick.

It's quite remote, in places. Some parts of the walk take us over well-trodden paths where your heart-attack will see you discovered and revived in mere minutes. Other sections are on *the path less travelled* (Frost,1920) such that when you are eventually found it will be no more than your bleached white bones which remain to decorate the scenery.

Taking the LZ702 to Femes, we park outside of the eponymous Femes Café. Where we will take coffee, now, and stew later while benefiting from clean toilets.

From the Church head uphill, passing the signed Mirador and turn Right onto a brick paved road. Pass along Calle Juan Caceres Martin, passing Calle Barranco Del Olivo following Camino de Los Pozos. The road curves away and we are following a cinder track around the mountain.

Soon the path offers us a turn on the Left which zig-zags up (and up) the mountain until finally emerging at the peak, near to telephone masts where the entire West coast is suddenly revealed, to dramatic effect. The view to the south is also dramatic, over onto the Playa Blanca plain. Near to the masts is a deserted house and a cave, which has indeed been developed as a dwelling, now abandoned. A very short way back down, we are offered a path on the Left that takes us to a second peak.

From here we would like to head East, to an oasis far below that hosts a roundabout and palm trees. The path there is not always clear but the landmark is always in sight so it presents little difficulty. Much of this part of the descent is in dry rivulets, over occasional dry walls and generally downwards, always facing the roundabout oasis.

If the fates favour us, we will see an artificial barranco ahead of us at right-angles to our travel. We slip into the barranco and follow it down (Right) to its end and there find ourselves at right angles to a path. We turn Left and the path widens out into a level area the purpose of which yet another Lanzarote mystery. Here the track ends. A path on a wall top sustains us for a short while but soon that, too, ends. From here, we can see another wall path down and to our left bordering onto a barranco. A very faint path will get us to it. From the bottom end of this second wall path we cross an abandoned vinyard and pass through a gateway onto the road. We travel on the tar macadam road for a very short way until we see a very deep storm drain which we enter and follow downhill, through a tunnel under the LZ702 and on. until it ends by a 40-foot shipping container.

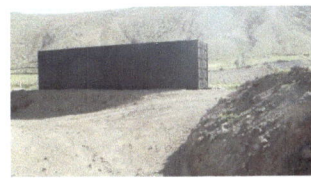

We must stop for a moment's admiration of the lorry driver who delivered the thing to this impossible location.

From the shipping container, we turn Right on a short track that becomes in turn a faint path on the top of a bank that a jeep track and finally a watercourse. The watercourse reaches a low concrete wall which we climb and continue forward along the watercourse which swings to our Right and following it we pass back under the LZ702, climb onto the pavement and trot back to the sanctuary of our car. Thankfully it is just outside the eponymous Café Femés, so toilets, beer and stew are immediately available as part of our celebration that we only took one of the short Femés walks. It could have been so much worse!

In the café, a familiar conversation emerges,

'Well of course walking for me is particularly difficult because one of my legs is shorter than the other'.

'One leg shorter than the other? That's nothing! One of mine is longer than the other and everyone knows that's much worse.'

Ha! A couple of mismatched legs is nothing; I've been walking for years with two arthritic hip joints'.

Only two arthritic joints? Luxury! I've had Arthritis, Rheumatism and Gout in every joint of my body for ninety-years and a broken ankle for the last ½-mile'.

'Arthritis, Rheumatism and Gout in every joint for ninety-years and a broken ankle. I long for such minor problems; you lot don't know what trouble is. I was born with no joints in my legs at all and had to ....'

Femés short West loop for Los Anciana

This is a 1-hour, circular, trainers walk, easy to find, without hard hill sections (or consequent restful descents) through easy terrain with reliable paths and clear direction. There's no risk of vertigo, and remarkable views of the settlement; this is a nice walk around the edge of a very charming town.

It is all on well-trodden paths where your heart-attack will see you discovered and revived in mere minutes. This is u our other walks on *the path less travelled* (Frost,1920) wherewhen you were eventually found it would be no more than your bleached white bones which remain to decorate the scenery.

Taking the LZ702 to Femes, we park outside of the eponymous Femes Café. Where we will take coffee, now, and stew later while benefiting from clean toilets.

From the Church head uphill, passing the Mirador and turn Right onto a brick road. Pass along Calle Juan Caceres Martin, passing Calle Barranco Del Olivo following Camino de Los Pozos. The road curves away and we are following a cinder track around the mountain.

Soon the path offers us a turn on the Left which zig-zags up (and up) the mountain. That is hard work, so don't do it! We follow the track gracefully around the mountain passing a few farmhouses and returning to tar macadam roads.

From here you could follow the road back to the car and more importantly the café Femes.

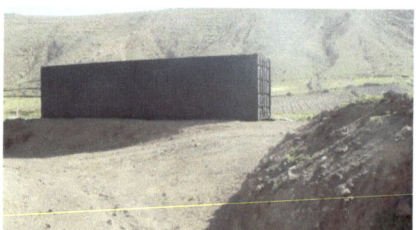

Alternatively we can avoid the road and extend our walk a little, thus:

We travel on the tar macadam road for a very short way until we see a very deep storm drain which we enter and follow downhill, passing through a tunnel under the LZ702, and on until it ends at a 40-foot shipping container.

We must stop for a moment to salute the lorry driver who delivered the thing to this impossible location.

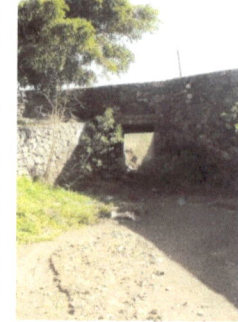

From the container, we turn Right on a short track that becomes a faint path on the top of a bank that becomes a track and finally a watercourse. The watercourse reaches a low concrete wall which we climb and continue forward along the watercourse which swings to our Right and following it we pass back under the LZ702 climb onto the pavement and trot back to the sanctuary of our car. Thankfully it is just outside the eponymous café Femes, so toilets beer and stew are immediately available as part of our celebration that we only took one of the short Femes walks. It could have been so much worse!

Femes long West loop

This is a 2½-hour, circular, trainers walk, mostly easy to find, with one or two hard hill sections followed by restful descents through rough terrain with unreliable paths but clear direction. There's no great risk of vertigo, and remarkable views of the South and West of the island. This is a nice walk around the edge of this very charming town. Take a compass, binoculars a map and your stick.

It's quite remote, in places. Some parts of the walk take us over well-trodden paths where your heart-attack will see you discovered and revived in mere minutes. Other sections are on *the path less travelled* (Frost,1920) such that when you are eventually found it will be no more than your bleached white bones which remain to decorate the scenery.

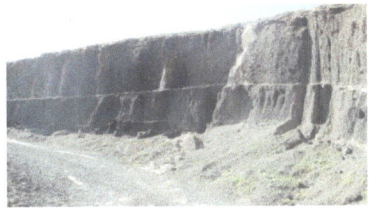

From the eponymous Femes Café, head uphill, passing the signed Mirador and turn Right onto a brick paved road. Pass along Calle Juan Caceres Martin, passing Calle Barranco Del Olivo following Camino de Los Pozos. The road curves away and we are following a cinder track around the mountain.

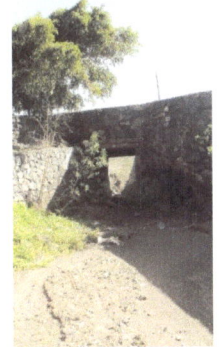

Soon the path offers us a turn on the right which zig-zags up (and up) the mountain until finally emerging at the peak, near to telephone masts where the entire West coast is suddenly revealed to fine effect. The view to the south is also dramatic, over onto the Playa Blanca plain.

This construction is worth attention. There are houses and caves that reward a few moments and offer respite.

A very short way back down, we are offered a path on the Left that takes us to a second peak. From here a fairly faint North-easterly path takes us down and then up to a second peak and then the same to a third, where a rough road will guide us on the next section.

We look for a sharp turning to the Right which guides us for a while and then peters out. From here we take a path South-East on the edge of the fields until it reaches a dirt track and thence the road. Trotting up the pavement we reach the bus shelter and then a storm drain crosses under the road. We drop down the steps into the drain, passing under the LZ702, and on until it ends at a 40-foot shipping container.

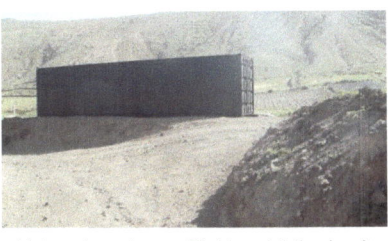

We salute the lorry driver who delivered the thing to this impossible location.

From the container, we turn Right on a short track that becomes a faint path on the top of a bank that becomes a track and finally a watercourse. The watercourse reaches a low concrete wall which we climb and continue forward along the watercourse which swings to our Right and following it we pass back under the LZ702 climb onto the pavement and trot back to the sanctuary of our car.

Thankfully it is just outside the eponymous Bar Femes, so toilets, beer and stew are immediately available as part of our celebration that it's all over. However we'll never understand why we undertook took one of the longest of the Femes walks. It could not have been much worse!

Goat to Goat, Femés

This is a 3-hour, circular, trainers walk, mostly easy to find, with one or two hard hill sections followed by restful descents through the most fantastic barranco we have yet found. There's no great risk of vertigo, and remarkable views of the South of the island. Take a compass, binoculars a map and your stick.

It's quite remote, in places. Some parts of the walk take us over well-trodden paths where your heart-attack will see you discovered and revived in mere minutes. Other sections are on *the path less travelled* (Frost,1920) such that when you are eventually found it will be no more than your bleached white bones which remain to decorate the scenery.

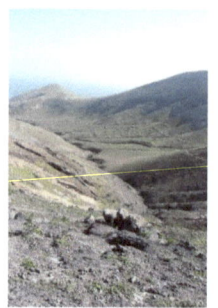

Taking the LZ702 to Femes, we park outside of the eponymous Café Femés. Where we will take coffee, now, and stew later while benefiting from clean toilets. On the opposite side of the LZ702 from the café we see a zig-zag track up to a building on the horizon.

This is a great goat farm, where we can mingle with these very fine animals if we wish. Dec – March we will see new-born goat kids all around us. From the peak, there are three paths to be seen. One winds its way around the high mountain to our Right; this is our return path. One follows the crest of the hill on our Left; this is the return from another walk, 'The Femes Barranco and Mountain Crest.'

We are taking the third path, which runs down into the valley. It is easy to see the paths in the distance, but difficult at the start as they are continually eroded by goats.

We scramble down and find the lowest of our three paths, and follow it through a magical valley over the water course until it forks and we select the Right path which will take us up to a mountain saddle, in another ½-hour or so. Lama Del Paso appears on out Left, and if masochism dictates it so, then we can make a short extra loop to experience the view from this peak.

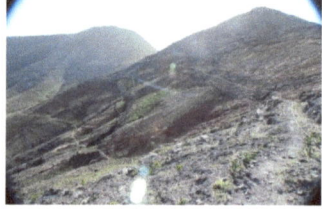

Paso excursion, or none, we continue until we are reassured to find a resting shelter where we might eat, drink and remove pecon from our shoes and shorts. The shelter is not in any way functional *(Affording no actual shelter)* and the decision to put it there is a complete mystery, but it serves very well to reassure us that we are on the correct path.

The path continues to wind around the mountain, affording an ever changing vista until in the pass between Pica Redondo and Hecha Grande we spy another goat farm to our left. We continue to follow the trail to the Right, traversing a path cut into the rock which also carries a black water pipe. The pipe serves to guide us all of the way back to the first goat farm. This is the water supply from one goat farm to the other. It is interesting to consider what a feat this installation was and also to speculate on just how hot the water must be when it arrives. Shower temperature for sure.

Pica Aceltuna (487-metres at the peak) is on our Left as we approach the original goat farm and if any spirit remains in us, we can climb to the top and look down onto the Femes Cafe, thinking just how good will be our post-perambulatory beer.

We return to the goat farm, pausing to once more enjoy the beauty of these graceful animals and then trot down the track to the Café. If you want, they will serve you goat stew. By now, we are realizing that there is little hope of a cure; our lot is to haunt the Lanzarotean landscape for ever more.

Valley and Ridge Circuit, Femés

This is a 3-hour, circular, trainers walk, only for the intrepid, not entirely easy to find, with one or two seriously hard hill sections after a delightful descent through the most fantastic barranco we have yet found. There's no great risk of vertigo, and remarkable views of the South of the island.

Not for a windy day! Take a compass, binoculars a map and your stick.

It's quite remote, in places. Some parts of the walk take us over well-trodden paths where your heart-attack will see you discovered and revived in mere minutes. Other sections are on *the path less travelled* (Frost,1920) such that when you are eventually found it will be no more than your bleached white bones which remain to decorate the scenery.

Taking the LZ702 to Femes, we park outside of the eponymous Bar Femés. Where we will take coffee, now, and stew later while benefiting from clean toilets.

On the opposite side of the LZ702 from the café we see a zig-zag track up to a building on the horizon.

This is a great fun goat farm, where we can mingle with these very fine animals if we wish. Dec – March we will even see new-born goat kids all around us.

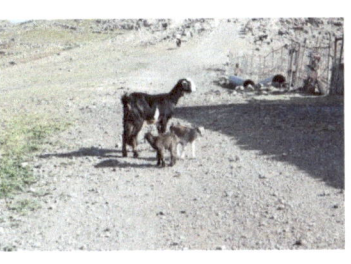

From the peak, there are three paths to be seen. One winds its way around the high mountain to our Right; one follows the crest of the hill on our Left; this is our return path.

We are taking the third path, which runs down into the valley. It is easy to see the paths in the distance, but difficult at the start as they are continually eroded by goats.

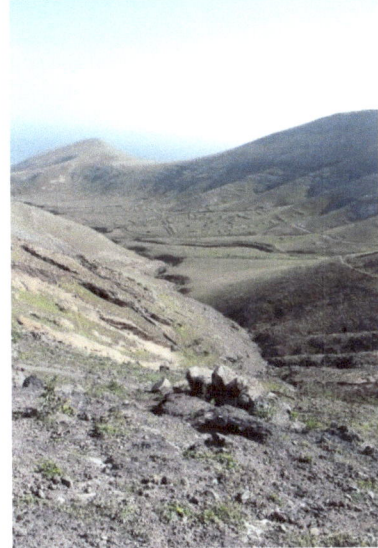

We scramble down and find the lowest of these three paths, and follow it through a magical valley over the water course until it forks and we pass by a turning on the Right path which would take us up to a mountain saddle and Lama Del Paso. We, however continue downwards.

We loop Left to cross a dry stream and then Right to reach a promontory. There is no real path but to the North-West we can see the peak of Pico Oveja and it is entirely possible to pick a path to that. Much panting and the burning of many calories brings us to the peak. Here we are rewarded by yet more fabulous viewing. A little to the West involving a degree of decent, we can reach the ridge. The path is not always clear, but it is reasonably easy to follow the crest of the ridge and eventually achieve the safety and comfort of the goat farm.

From here, we can drop down to the eponymous bar and steady ourselves with beer and stew. You, I know, are going to wonder why *(oh why?)* you do it, but I am afraid that I am unable to help you with that. It makes no sense to me either.

Montana Cuervo

This is a 1-hour, trainers, walk, not remotely strenuous, with no risk of vertigo. Fabulous to experience the inside of a volcano.

This is coach-potato country – not at all remote. A well-trodden path where your heart-attack will see you discovered and revived in mere minutes. It is beloved of coach parties, so selecting the best time of day is important but the gap in the corona that admits you onto the floor of the volcano is one of the best.

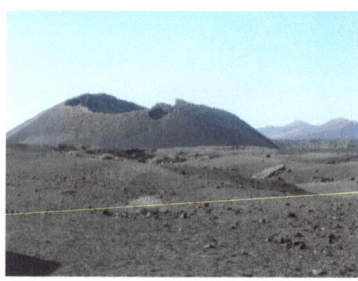

We take the LZ30, which runs from Teguise to Mozaga and on towards Uga and near to Masdache we take the LZ56, North, for a very short way until we see a large car park on our left.

A very good path has been created to take us to the volcano and it is clear and easy to find. When we reach the mountain we can turn left or right, circumnavigating the mountain in either clockwise or anticlockwise direction. Each is as good as the other, but note that the entrance to the volcano is a short way to our right. Whether we want to get there now or later rather depends on which is least likely to see us coinciding with a coach party. The good thing is that the coach trip sees people rush in, photograph each other and rush out again as quickly as possible to reach the next shop on their itinerary. So, with a little patience we can always get this mystical enclosure to ourselves and such is the ambience inside the mountain that we really do want to be alone there.

The walk around the volcano is really very engaging and needs regular stops just to marvel. The path takes us into lava fields that are as good as we would find anyway and very easily accessed - unlike some to which we might take you.

Having communed with ourselves inside the volcano, gazing up at high mountain walls, and walked through fine volcanic lava fields, we reach our return track. From here, there is a clear path up to the corona which is quite inviting, but vertigo cannot be ruled out and the signs clearly do not encourage this climb so we will not either.

If it was just me, I'd go straight on to climb Montana Negra, now, leaving the car where it is and doing enough puffing and panting to feel that I'd had a respectable day of exercise. From that fine mountain peak there is a fabulous view down onto Montana Cuervo.

If that's too much for you, there is a fine Sociodad in Mancha Blanca. However, that being the case, I will not want to hear grumbles. This was not a walk enough to raise a sweat.

Montana Negra

This is a 1½ -hour, trainers, walk, pretty strenuous, but with only minimal risk of vertigo in spite of a 515-m peak height. Fabulous views over the volcanoes of the South and a remarkable view down onto the famous Montana Cuervo. Take a compass, binoculars a map and your stick.

Quite remote. Some walks take us over well-trodden paths where your heart-attack will see you discovered and revived in mere minutes. We love this one, though, because it takes us on *the path less Travelled* and when you are eventually found it will be no more than your bleached bones that remain to decorate the scenery.

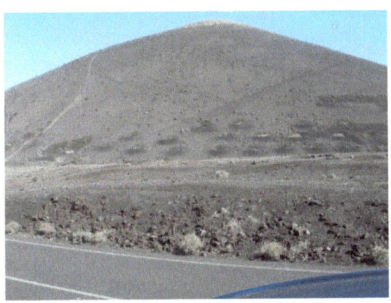

We take the LZ30, which runs from Teguise to Mozaga and on towards Uga and near to Masdache we take the LZ56, North, for a very short way until we see a large car park on our left.

Our mountain is on the right and we can see the path options running to the mountain peak.

Walking to the mountain path is simple and we start our ascent next to a building that is still in use for agricultural purposes. We struggle upwards along a path that keeps forking and dividing. This is a good, literal, example of 'Many roads up the mountain' and it doesn't really matter which we choose. Each goes to the same place. Some circle the mountain gently and some ascend rather more directly and each is fine as long as we select one that is generally uphill. After a while we reach the bowl of the volcano, and the general greenery in the bowl is quite remarkable.

Like so many mountains here, it suddenly becomes quite lush and verdant. This greenery continues right to the peak. In autumn, the sedums are in flower, as are the geraniums and later the marguerites making this a colourful spot. There is also a decent grove of olive trees. From here two 'arms' reach up to the peak. Either arm makes a satisfactory route uphill. From the peak, we can look down on the Montana Cuervo and beyond it to a vast array of mountains in all directions. A while with a map and compass will see us identifying mountains and habitations all around.

Descent, when we are ready again can be conducted in many directions, noticing Caldera Colorada just to our North.

Were it me, I would now trot over and try Caldera Colorada, but if you prefer then it's a Post-perambulatory cold beer at the Sociodad in Mancha Blanca, where you might swear never to attempt Colorada, but we both know you'll weaken, and give it a go.

Montana Colorada

This is a 1-hour, trainers, walk, not remotely strenuous, with no risk of vertigo. Fine way to see a 'Bomb' and read up on the making of a volcano.

This is coach-potato country – not at all remote. Well-trodden path where your heart-attack will see you discovered and revived in mere minutes. Beloved of coach parties, so selecting the best time of day is important but the walk is pleasant and the explanations of the volcano is one of the best.

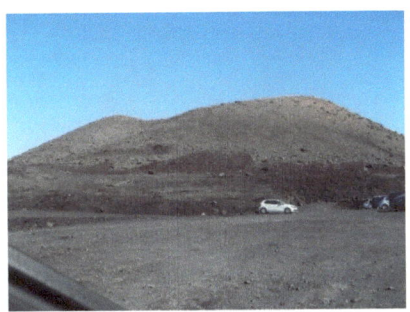

We take the LZ30, which runs from Teguise to Mozaga and on towards Uga, and near to Masdache we take the LZ56, North, a short way until we see a large car park on our left. Our mountain is a little further on the right again with a car park.

We can walk either clockwise or anticlockwise and there is no benefit to either, save that we can avoid a crowd by choosing whichever option they eschew.

Throughout the National Park walks we find photographs, maps (usually incorrectly orientated) and descriptions of landscape that would embarrass even a geography teacher. This landscape it the most dramatic, exciting, thrilling, stirring, stimulating, inspiring, electrifying and motivating scenery we could ever hope to find. *(And I only end there because my stock of synonyms is so limited.)* However, *the powers* have a way of writing copy to make the most exciting vision ever seem duller than the worst geography lesson you ever slept through. Perhaps it's better in the original Spanish. Anyway, the boards on this walk are the exception so allow time to look at them. They explain the creation of a bomb, meaning a rock that congealed in the sky and fell to ground, leaving you grateful if you were standing somewhere else. Near the sign is an excellent example of the phenomenon.

Further around, the creation of a volcanic corona is explained. You will have noticed that most of the volcanoes face in the same direction. *(If you haven't, then look around you now.)* Nearly all have a high 'head' and a pair of 'arms', curling around towards a large gap, looking faintly like a cartoon character. All point in one direction and that is because much of the corona is formed from pitched ash and this is affected by prevailing winds and… Anyway, if you read the explanations, this will all be made clear to you.

While walking, you will see a path slanting up through the pecon to the corona. This is a worthwhile effort affording a fine view of the inside of the volcano and also of the Montana Negra, behind you. However, this is a tough climb, the ground under foot not as firm as you'd like and vertigo a serious issue. So, if you pass that by, that's probably wise.

Having walked full circle, you will have had a pleasant stroll. If you're now ready for a climb, scramble up Montana Negra, next door.

If not Negra, then it's a Post-perambulatory cold beer at the Sociodad in Mancha Blanca, where you might swear never to attempt Negra, but we both know you'll weaken, eventually, and give it a go.

Montana Los Rodeos

This is a 2-hour, trainers, Near-circular walk, not very strenuous, with no risk of vertigo, even on the optional 454-m peak height. Fabulous views over the volcanoes of the South and a remarkable stretch of lava.Take a compass, binoculars a map and your stick.

Quite remote. Some walks take us over well-trodden paths where your heart-attack will see you discovered and revived in mere minutes. We love this one, though, because it takes us on *the path less Travelled* and when you are eventually found it will be no more than your bleached bones that remain to decorate the scenery.

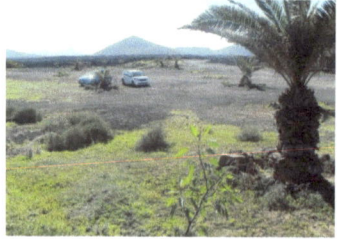

Park in the delightful oasis towards the North end of the LZ56, Just to the South of Mancha Blanca.

Walk along the left of the paths, which is the one not stone surfaced and soon you will be puzzled by a hobbit hole in the hill on your right. This is a block structure and although this is an extensive construction it only actually encloses a space big enough to park a car. Perhaps the rest of the structure is to give protection against rocks and water tumbling from the mountain.

Continuing along this path takes us through some impressive and very varied lava fields. In places looking as though it has just run, cooled and set yesterday.

The path is a good one, progressing steadily to the mountain. At the base of the mountain we are able to turn left or right. Each is

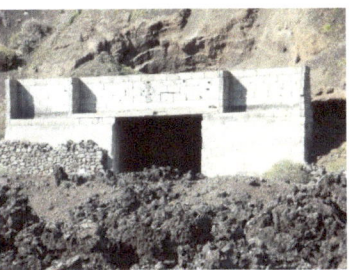

as good as the other so if there should be other walkers, we always take the route that ensures the greatest solitude.

Anyway, turn left or right *as you like* and process around this double-peaked mountain. Offered further forks, we just take the route that holds us closest to the mountain.

This is another twin-peaked mountain and when we are at the furthest point in our circuit we can climb to the lower and thence to the higher peak. Not too tough in the main and it gives us a magical view.

From the high peak there is an option *(I'm afraid)*. We could retrace our steps to the far end of the circuit and continue our mountain circumnavigatory route. This is probably a good option as the lava is varied and well worth seeing. Alternatively, though, this peak is the volcano's 'head' and the usual two 'arms' curve out to the North and it is perfectly possible to walk down either of these arms to the ground and we find ourselves at the original and philosophically troublesome T-junction, with just one section of track left to travel before returning to the blessed sanctuary which is our car.

From the car, the nearest cold beer is in Mancha Blanca at the Sociodad. Sat in the bar we wonder why we did not just park in the lovely oasis, take a few snaps, and have a little nap in the car. *Maybe next time; nobody will know.*

Uga short Loop

This is a 1½ -hour, almost-circular, trainers walk, easy to find, with one long hard hill climb through fine grape country, followed by good views and a restful descent. There's no risk of vertigo, in spite of a 507-Metre peak, and remarkable views of the vineyards and the myriad mountains of the South.

It's not remote, but a pleasantly quiet track. May still be bleached white bones territory, in places. From the LZ206, driving West, take the LZ30, North and park at the footpath, signed on your right in a few hundred metres.

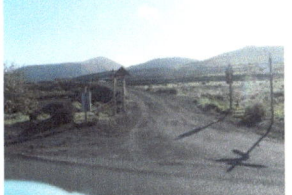

We park near the entrance to the track. This is a section of the Orzola to Playa Blanca route, so adequately signed. It is also intensively farmed, so the road is pretty good.

Head eastwards and upwards, through vine basins and fig trees.

The road is raised a good height in place for no reason that I can identify.

And up, and up, *(and up)* pausing regularly to draw breath and feign interest the endless vineyards across the valley we remember how much good this is doing us. In the autumn, the figs are abundant and although small are absolutely delicious. Most are left to rot as you will see by looking at the ground under the three, so I feel OK about scrumping a few. However, they can have an unwelcome effect for one so far from a toilet, so for myself I am modest in my sampling. As we get, thankfully, near to the top three car tracks appear on the right and after those a foot path on the right

Following the path steeply upwards we strike a jeep track, which we can follow around to our Right, to reach a first, a second (higher) and a third (highest) peak, each offering a different fine view.

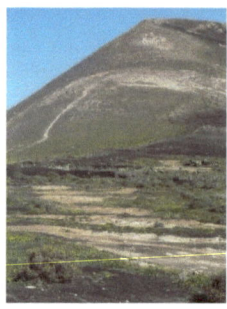

Recovered and refreshed, our track loops on around to the left passing a complex of al jibes and a ruin before finally regaining our original road/track at the mountain pass. From here, the view is East as well as West so different again.

Across the track, you might be tempted by the near-perfect cone of Montana de Guardilama. This is a steep path, with a mild risk of vertigo and will take about an extra 40-mins, but the view is fab and otherwise our walk from here is a gently downhill trek to the refuge of

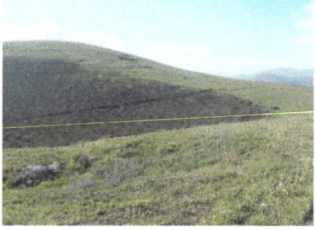

the car, so maybe it is OK to go.

From here, having popped up to the peak and back *(or not – nobody will judge you)* we take the track back to the West, towards Uga and the safe haven which is our car. This is a very gentle coasting down all of the way and takes remarkably little time. Do pause, though, to look in detail at the ever-changing view across the valley and Uga nestled between the hills. Notice a very odd circular hole surrounded by a smart wall in the centre of Uga. You will probably want to know what it is and my answer is *'So do I'*. Later, if we follow signs to the Mercado we will find this excavation and a careful study will leave us none-the-wiser.

Attaining the protection afforded us by our car, Uga is clearly the nearest source of post-perambulatory (purely medicinal) alcohol. Even for me, Mala and the Arepera are too far to go. So in Uga, we eat, drink remove pecon from\intimate places and congratulate ourselves on selecting the shortest of the three Uga walks.

Uga Loop

This is a 2½ -hour, circular, trainers walk, easy to find, with one long hard hill climb through fine wine country, followed by good views and a restful descent. There's no risk of vertigo, in spite of a 507-Metre peak and there are remarkable views of the vineyards and the myriad mountains of the South.

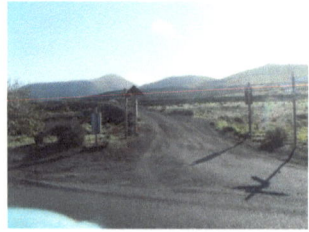

From the LZ206, driving West, take the LZ30, North and park at the footpath, signed on your right in a few hundred metres.

We park near the entrance to the track. This is a section of the Orzola to Playa Blanca route, so adequately signed. It is also intensively farmed, so the road is pretty good.

Head eastwards and upwards, through vine basins and fig trees.

It is interesting to study the stone walls giving wind protection to the vines. These are totally frail, single stones, one on another and look entirely fragile. The nature of the volcanic rock is such that it just locks together and lasts for ever. The pods on the beach are the same, of course. The road is raised a good height in place for no reason that I can identify.

And up, and up, pausing regularly to gaze at the endless vineyards across the valley and remember how much good this is doing us. In Autumn, the figs are abundant and although small are absolutely delicious. Most are left to rot as you will see by looking at the ground under the three, so I feel OK about sampling a few. However, they can have an unfortunate effect for one so far from a toilet, so for myself I am cautious.

After much effort and no little perspiration, we reach the mountain pass and are rewarded by fabulous Easterly views. Here, however, we have a cunning plan for adding still more climbing to our route! We will take the jeep track on our Right between two low stone pillars. Circling South and looping around to our Right, passing the ubiquitous ruined farm and a complex set of al jibes we reach the mountain's peak (Montana Tinasaria). Here, we pause to eat, drink, curse the pecon in our shoes, and enjoy the view.

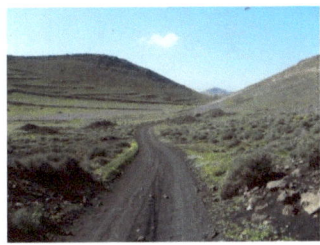 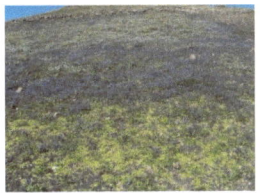 Head on, downwards along the track for just a short way we reach another slight plateau. From here we can see an (only mildly precipitous) track down the side of the mountain to join a jeep track that heads West. Following the jeep track, we pass between fine mountains and emerge to gain a good view of Uga and our destination.

Occasionally in the winter, this route can display a continuous mass of flowers, resembling a wild-flower meadow.

Continuing, we see a strange concrete structure on the hill to our left, which turns out to be the run-off for another failed reservoir. The position should allow for collection of a great deal of water; the positioning is perfect and the catchment area extensive. However the rock is porous and we can see from the vegetation that it has never held water; not even for a short period. Reaching the road, we turn Right and walk, uphill, to the safety of the car.

Uga is the nearest source of post-perambulatory (purely medicinal) alcohol. Even for me, Mala and the Arepera would be too far to go. Eat, drink and congratulate yourselves on selecting the second shortest of the three Uga walks.

Uga long Loop

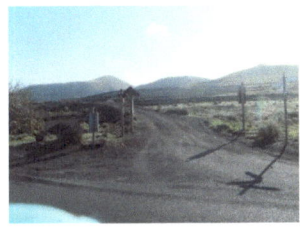 This is a 3½ -hour, circular, trainers walk, easy to find, with one long hard hill climb through fine country, followed by good views and a restful descent. *(OK, and a few more slight climbs)*. There's no risk of vertigo, in spite of a 507-Metre peak and remarkable views of the vineyards and the myriad mountains of the South.

It's not remote, but a pleasantly quiet track. May still be bleached white bones territory, in places, though.

From the LZ206, driving West, take the LZ30, North and park at the footpath, signed on your right in a few hundred metres.

We park near the entrance to the track. This is a section of the Orzola to Playa Blanca route, so adequately signed. It is also intensively farmed, so the road is pretty good.

Head eastwards and upwards, through vine basins and fig trees. We study the stone walls giving wind protection to the vines. These appear totally frail, single stones, one on another and look entirely fragile. The nature of the volcanic rock is such, though, that it just locks together and lasts for ever. The pods on the beach are the same, of course. The road is raised a good height in places, also for no reason that I can identify.

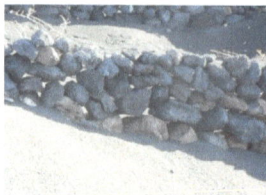 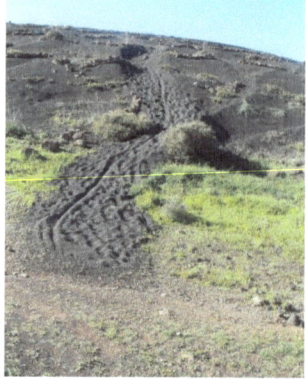

And up, and up, pausing regularly to gaze at the endless vineyards across the valley and remember how much good this is doing us. In Autumn, the figs are abundant and although small are absolutely delicious. Most are left to rot as you will see by looking at the ground under the three, so I feel OK about sampling a few. However, they can have an unfortunate effect for one so far from a toilet, so for myself I am modest in my scrumping.

As we get, thankfully, near to the top three car tracks appear on the right and after those a path on the right.

Following the path steeply upwards we strike a jeep track, which we can follow around, to reach a first, a second and a third peak, each offering a different fine view.

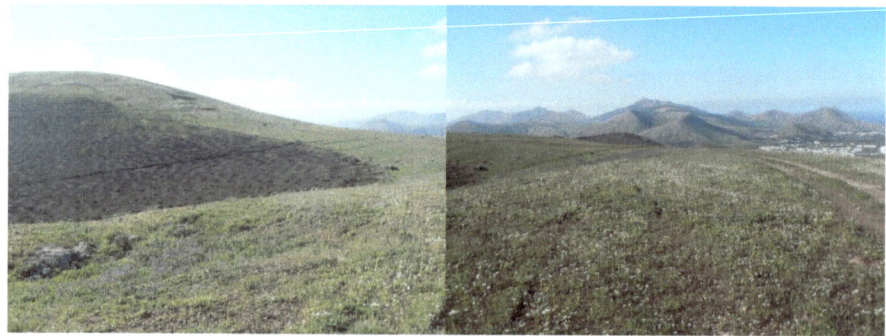

Recovered and refreshed, our track loops on around to the left passing a complex of al jibes and a ruin before finally regaining our original road/track on the mountain pass. From here, the view is East, so different again.

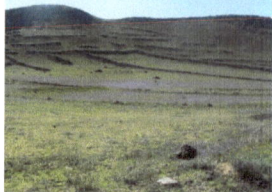

Now, we head on East, downhill passing a farm entrance and then turning right to head towards the sea. On our left we are passing some of the best gardens to be seen on the island. On our right we are impressed to see a small football area with real grass.

Onwards and downwards, we reach a cross-road and turn Right. We pass a mass of al jibes. Each has a large concrete water collecting area, rather than a channel to catch the mountain run-off. Were there contest for the most al jibes per acre, this would surely take it.

Just before reaching a roundabout, near the signpost, we strike off to the right on a jeep track that follows a line of pylons. It feels good to be away from the tar macadam again. We pass an isolated farm with a busy windmill, and continue on *(and on)* until we reach a cross-road. Here we turn Right, pushing uphill to reach a mountain pass where we swing Left. Following this track, we pass through

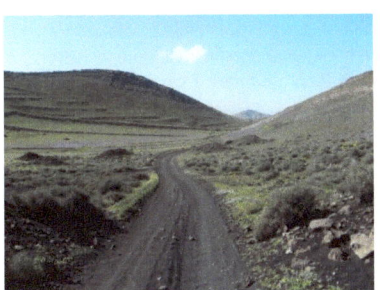

and between several mountains to emerge into what can be a charming flower meadow in a wet autumn/spring. There is a pleasant little volcano on our right worthy of a slight detour although the basin is not deep.

Continuing, we see a strange concrete structure on the hill to our Left which turns out to be the run-off for another failed reservoir. The position should allow for

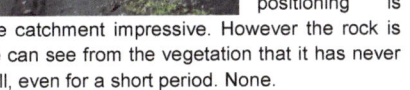

collection of a great deal of water; the positioning is

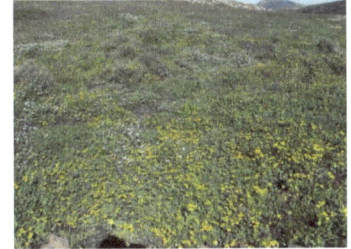

perfect and the catchment impressive. However the rock is porous and we can see from the vegetation that it has never held water at all, even for a short period. None.

Reaching the road, we turn Right and walk, uphill, to grasp the emotional crutch which is our car.

Uga is the nearest source of post-perambulatory (purely medicinal) alcohol. Even for me, Mala and the Arepera is too far to go. Eat, drink and commiserate with yourselves on selecting the longest of the three Uga walks. Still, at least it has finished.

Caldera Caldereta and Blanca

This is a 2½-hour, hard soled, walk, not especially strenuous, with some (optional) risk of vertigo on a 460-m high corona. Fabulous views across the national park. Take a compass, binoculars and your stick.

This is a walk down a well-trodden, official path so your heart-attack will see you discovered and revived in mere minutes. A not entirely easy walk you do have to work at it in places. Not this time, 'the path less Travelled' (Frost,1920) where when you were eventually found it would be no more than your bleached bones that remain to decorate the scenery.

We park in Mancha Blanca, on a westerly track off the LZ67, where there are several official parking spaces, just North-East of the Visitor's Centre. We take the obvious westerly path, reading dull explanations of lava along the way. The lava is spectacular and ever-changing and worth the walk all on its own. How it is that 'The Authorities' manage to make the information boards so desperately dull is a mystery. They are informative in the manner adopted by the very worst geography lessons you ever experienced. The path is good, wide and clear but stony so hard soles and a stick are a must. Frequently we see an interesting lava feature and must allow time to marvel at it all as well as just paying photographic homage.

The path is a bit too good and we fear the coach potato, but fear not; it becomes difficult, unclear and slightly dangerous before long, so our sense of adventure will be more than sated.

The path first reaches; a smaller mountain at just 326-metres, but fabulous. It is possible to scramble up the scree to the corona but not essential because there is more to come. Rounding the volcano, we see that there is a 'ground-level' entrance to the volcanic bowl with al jibes and ruins at the entrance. It is essential to round the bolder and walk into this bowl. Stand in the centre and rotate, for full effect. This may be one of our favourite volcano basins. Exiting the Caldereta entrance, we notice a sort of bridge in front of us and inspection shows that it is covering another al jibe and one so efficient as to be usually full, even after many years of neglect.

Our path requires us to walk gently upwards along the side of the Caldereta and once we are about half way up the side we see that the path strike off to our right through lava. *(Again, we use the term path rather loosely.)* The trick is to remember that we are heading for Blanca and pick our way forward. Sometimes there is no path at all and then we suddenly stumble upon a clearly pathified section. This *path – no path* section takes us over lava quite unlike that which we saw earlier and soon drops us onto a real path where we turn right(ish) before, by a huge boulder, we see a path diagonally up the side of the Caldera Blanca itself.

Climbing to the corona is achieved by way of a clearly visible path, which occasionally makes use of a water channel such that we are walking in a 1-metre deep trench. Broaching the corona we are treated to the most impressive view into the bowl ahead of us and behind us another view over many miles. Those who experience vertigo can enjoy this very wide ledge and its unthreatening views and take a picnic at this point. The map&compass come into play here, identifying towns and mountains all around us before we send the vertigo sufferers back down the path to the sanctuary of a collection of inexplicable corrals from where it is possible to turn Right and rejoin the outbound path. Retrace to the car.

Less sensitive souls can navigate the corona either way around; both are possible. We then drop down a steep 'path' at the Westernmost point to the base of the mountain and take a path North and then East to gain the sanctuary of the collection of inexplicable corrals mentioned above. From there it is possible to continue East and rejoin the outbound path at the al jibe we saw when exiting Caldereta.

Retracing our steps we achieve the sanctuary that we have missed since so foolishly leaving the car. The nearest restorative bar is in Mancha Blanca, which also boasts a supermarket if our water has been exhausted.

Montana Ubigue, Nazaret - for the timid

This is a 1½-hour, trainer, walk, not especially strenuous, with no risk of vertigo on a 308-m high corona. Nice views across Nazaret and Tahiche and the mountains to the West.

Take Map&Compass and your binoculars.

This is a walk up and down a jeep path so your heart-attack will see you discovered and revived in mere minutes. Not this time, *'the path less Travelled'* (Frost,1920) where when you were eventually found it would be no more than your bleached white bones that remain to decorate the scenery.

An entirely easy walk over clear tracks and on an old corona that is greatly softened by time. There are no rocky outcrops; no precipitous slopes. Good for the timid who still want to look down from the corona. You do have to work in the initial climb, but after that it's a coast.

We take the LZ10, South fromTeguise and just before it reaches a left-hand bend with protective rails, we take a road on the right. We follow that road into Nazaret over a cross road and as it deteriorates we find an informal parking area on the right, bordered with boulders.

We continue walking along this road, forking Left, signed casa Nazaret. We pass a farmhouse and the track dips to pass through a gulley with an ornate bridge to our Right. The purpose of this bridge is a mystery, if you know the answer, *(Gunga Din),* then you are a better man than I. The path continues; we ignore a fork to our Left (our return route) pass the barranco and see a jeep track running up the side of the mountain.

> *(Personally, I'd not take my Morris Minor up that track but as we keep seeing Lanzarotean drivers take vehicles to the most unlikely places.)*

The climb is a bit of a puff, but that is why it does us so much good. We reach the first peak and the view to the Left of mountains Zanzamas and Maneje are very pleasing. We progress to the higher peak, marked with a cross. From here the view of Tahiche and beyond to Costa Teguise are good or in the other direction, over Nazaret. To the left we see the volcano's basin and the barranco.

Refreshed, watered, fed and relieved of intrusive pecon, we can make our way down the second arm of this volcano, still following the jeep track. This rejoins our earlier route and we recognise the turning that we passed earlier. The track gently returns to the car. Having had such an easy outing so far you might want to run this last bit *(not!)*.

Returning, there are ample bars for post-perambulatory beer and tapas, but we prefer to experience delayed gratification by waiting until we reach Mala and The Arepera *. In whichever bar we sit, it behoves us to applaud each-other for the wisdom displayed in selecting such a nice short walk.

> ** I guide like this you when you are faced with a choice, each option having equal benefit, lest you find yourself unable to decide. In a deterministic universe, we imagine that we have free-will, but in fact all actions are determined by that which has gone before. So, we will make a left/right (yes/no, up/down, etc) decision based on our set of experiences to date. Since we have only one past (one make-up and one set of experiences) we can make only one decision at any time and any sense we have of 'free-will' is illusory. What we will do in any situation is 'predetermined' by what has happened before. An interesting consequence of this is that if we have no relevant experience, then we may be unable to decide at all. Determinism dictates that a donkey equidistant between two identical feed mangers will be unable to favour one over the other, unable to decide, and will starve to death. (Of course, this is a thought experiment; no real donkey involved. Like Schrödinger's cat; no cat was rendered simultaneously alive and dead just to demonstrate quantum theory) (For a full explanation of quantum theory and how it clashes with general relativity, see app'x 1).*
>
> *You, faced with two equal choices and no information to guide you may prove ill-equipped to make a decision.*

Thank you

Thank you for coming with us. We've had you in mind at every step and we really do feel your company on each walk. Write to us: nwheeler@brookes.ac.uk

And remember, if you feel that you would like to take more walks with Lambert and Wheeler, there are people at your Local Health Centre who can cure that. Otherwise, when the urge strikes to take a Lambert and Wheeler walk just lie down in a darkened room and it will pass off.

www.ingramcontent.com/pod-product-compliance
Lightning Source LLC
Chambersburg PA
CBHW050926290526

45792CB00002B/895